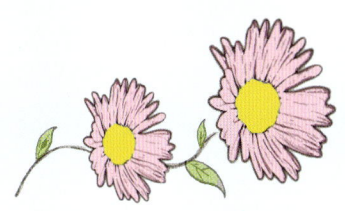

This Book is Dedicated to:

Kids who want to be well
&
Stay well

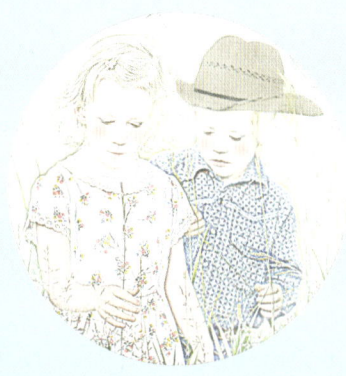

A portion of the proceeds from the sale of this book
will fund the improvement of health care for children around the world.

ISBN: 978-0-9980308-6-9
Little Me And You Books LLC
Leo Paper 2020
Manufactured in China

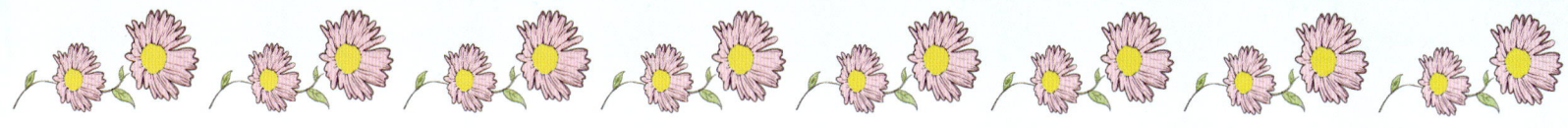

Little Me & You Books

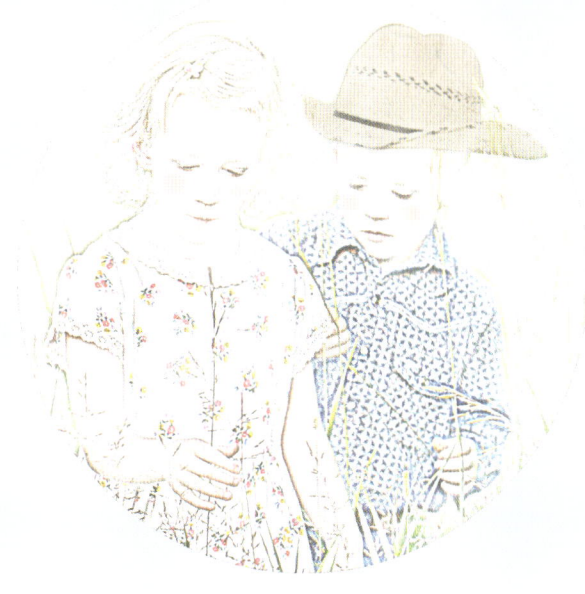

Healthy Me Collection
Book 1

Written & Illustrated by Lisa Kack

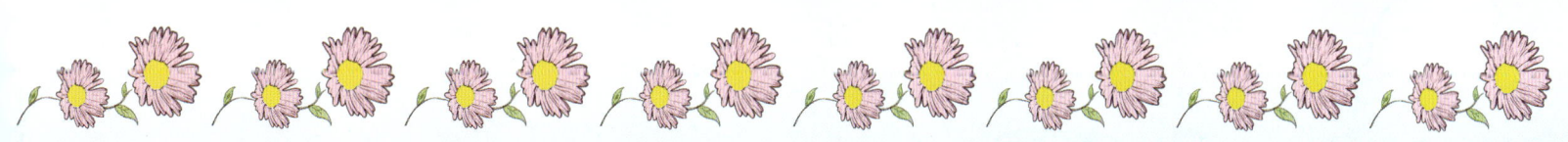

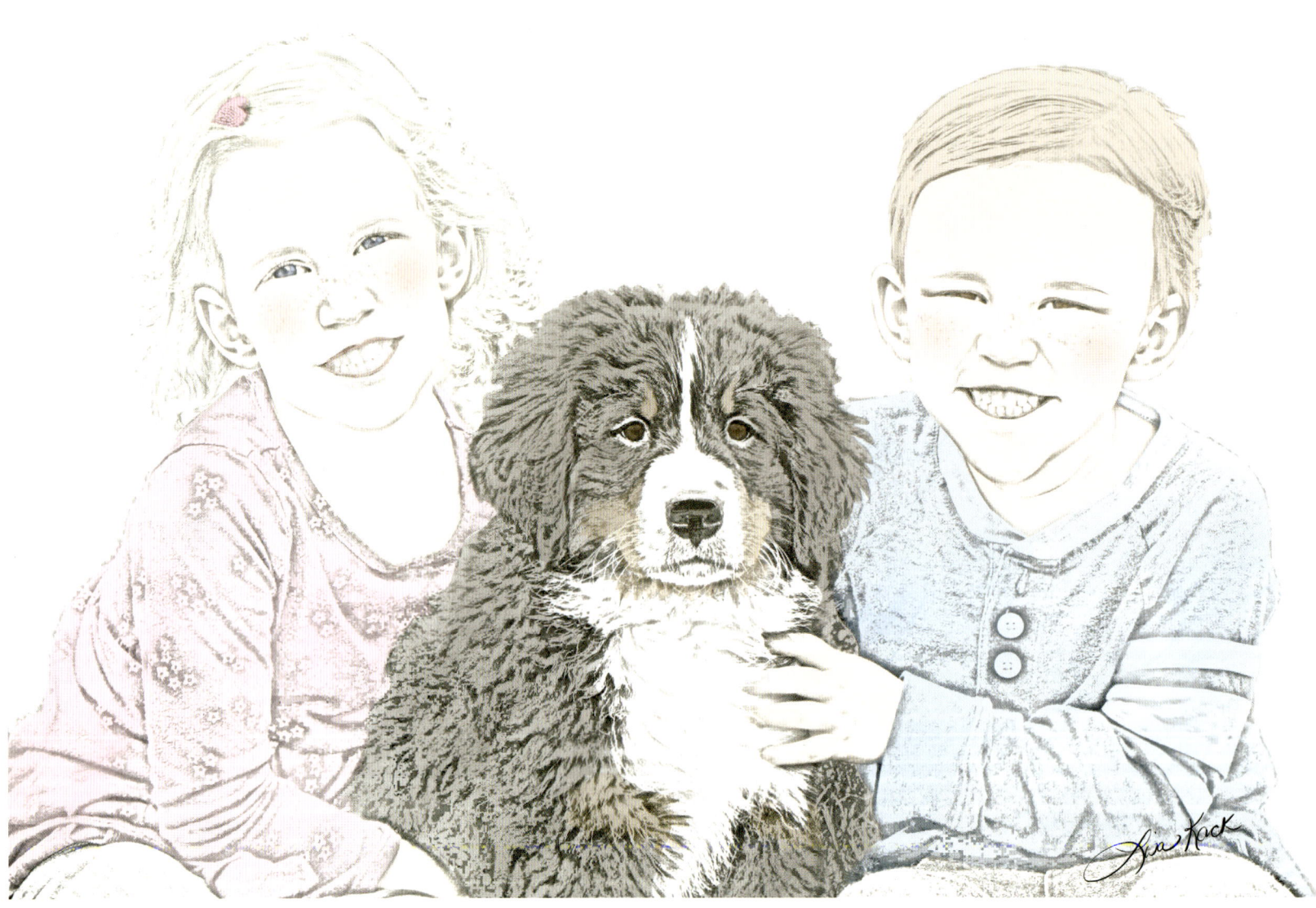

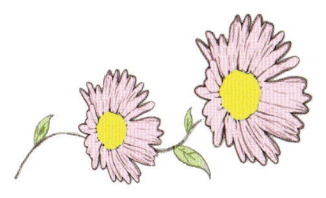

There are 10 important things

That boys and girls can do

To be a Healthy Little Me

And chase the sick bugs, too.

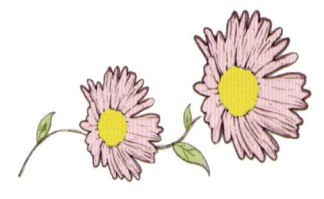

The first and most important

Is to wash my hands.

I scrub and scrub before each meal,

After using the toilet,

And after blowing my drippy nose.

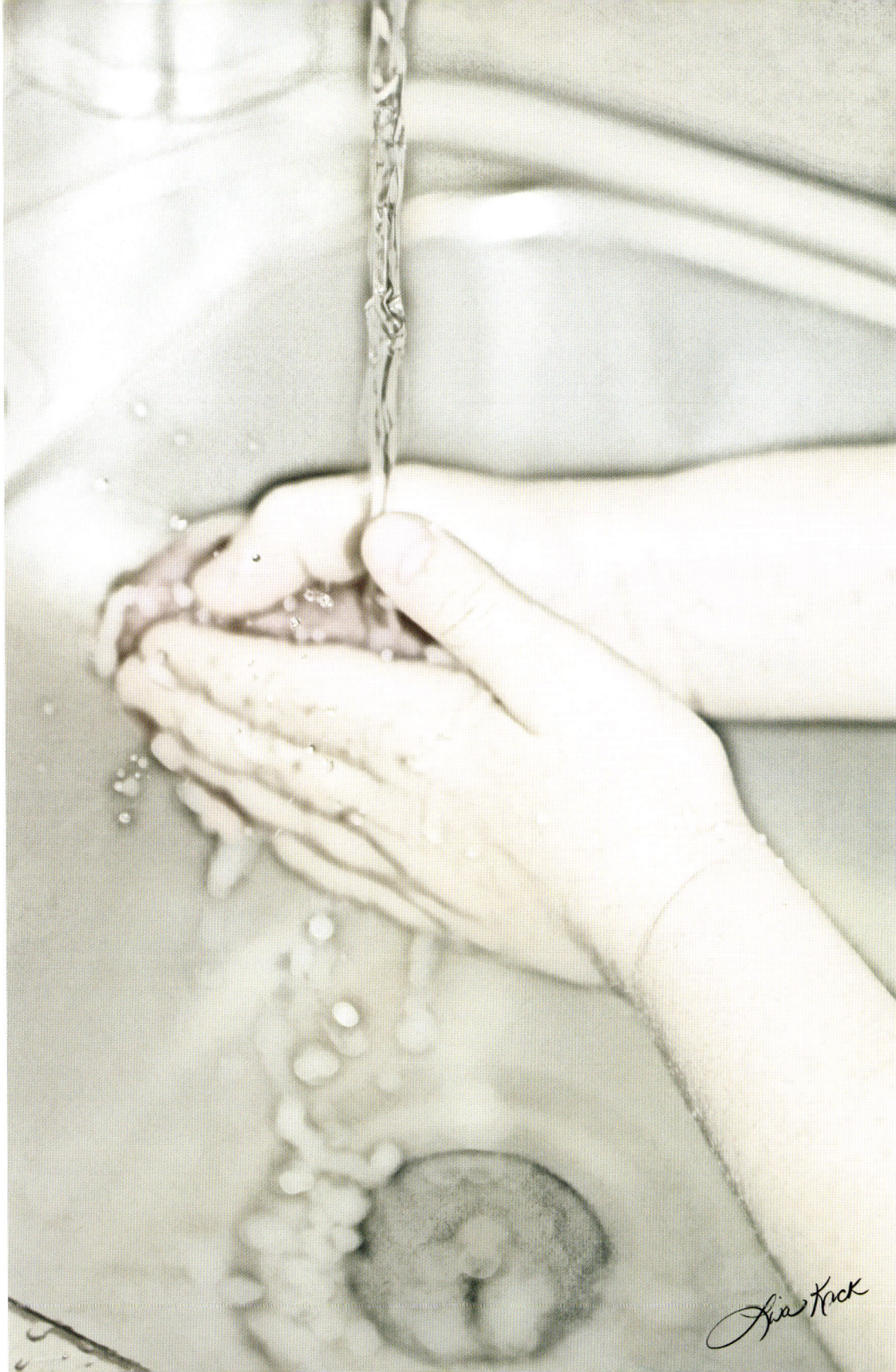

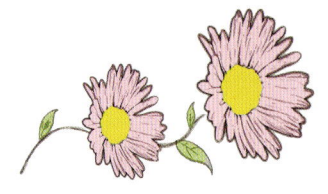

When I wake up in the morning,

I put on nice clean clothes.

I stay smelling fresh all through the day

And keep dirty sweat bugs

Washed away!

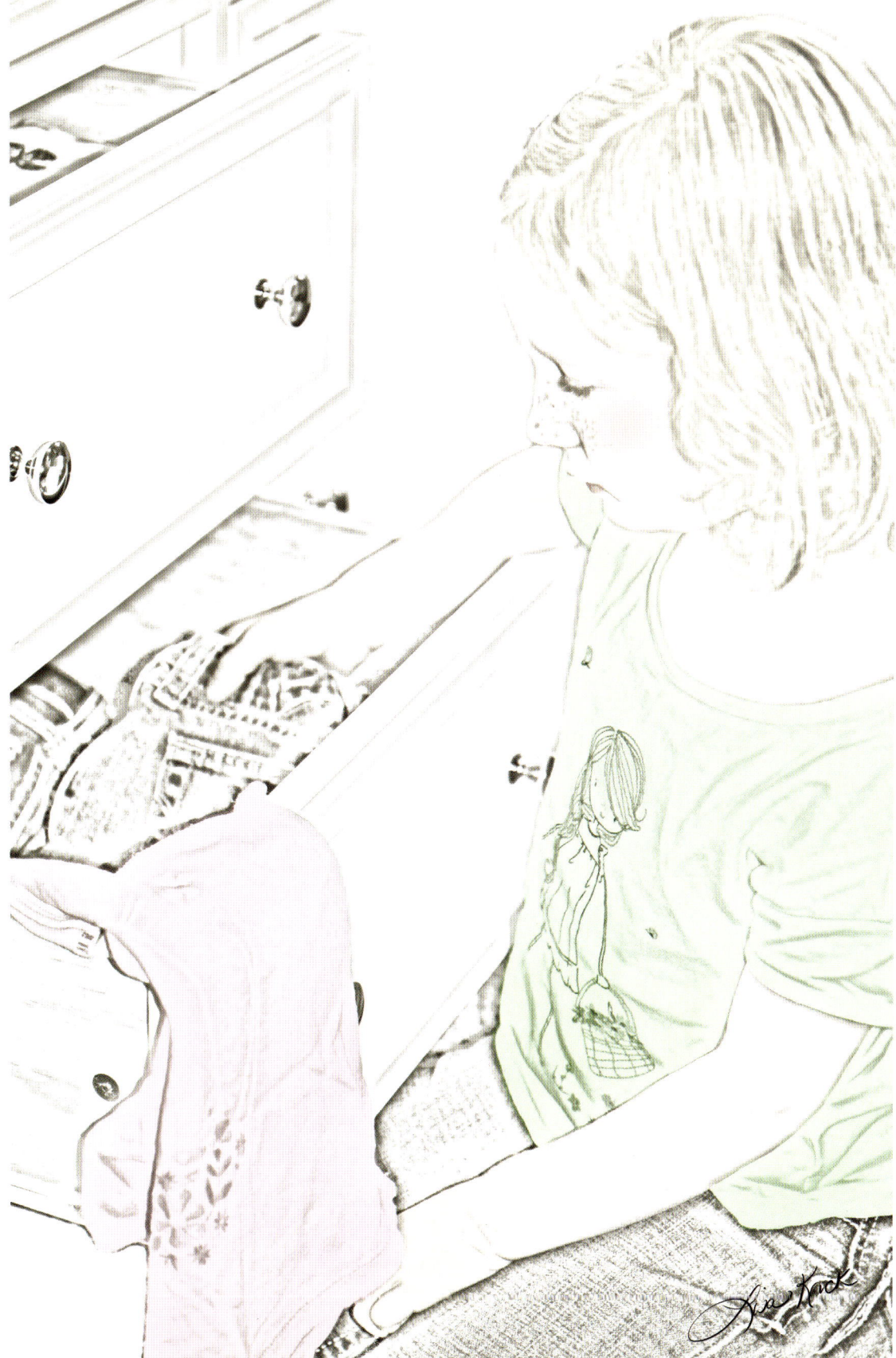

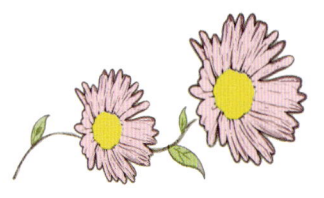

Every day I take a bath

To scrub the dirt away.

The bubbles wash the bad things out

And leave me squeaky clean -

No doubt!

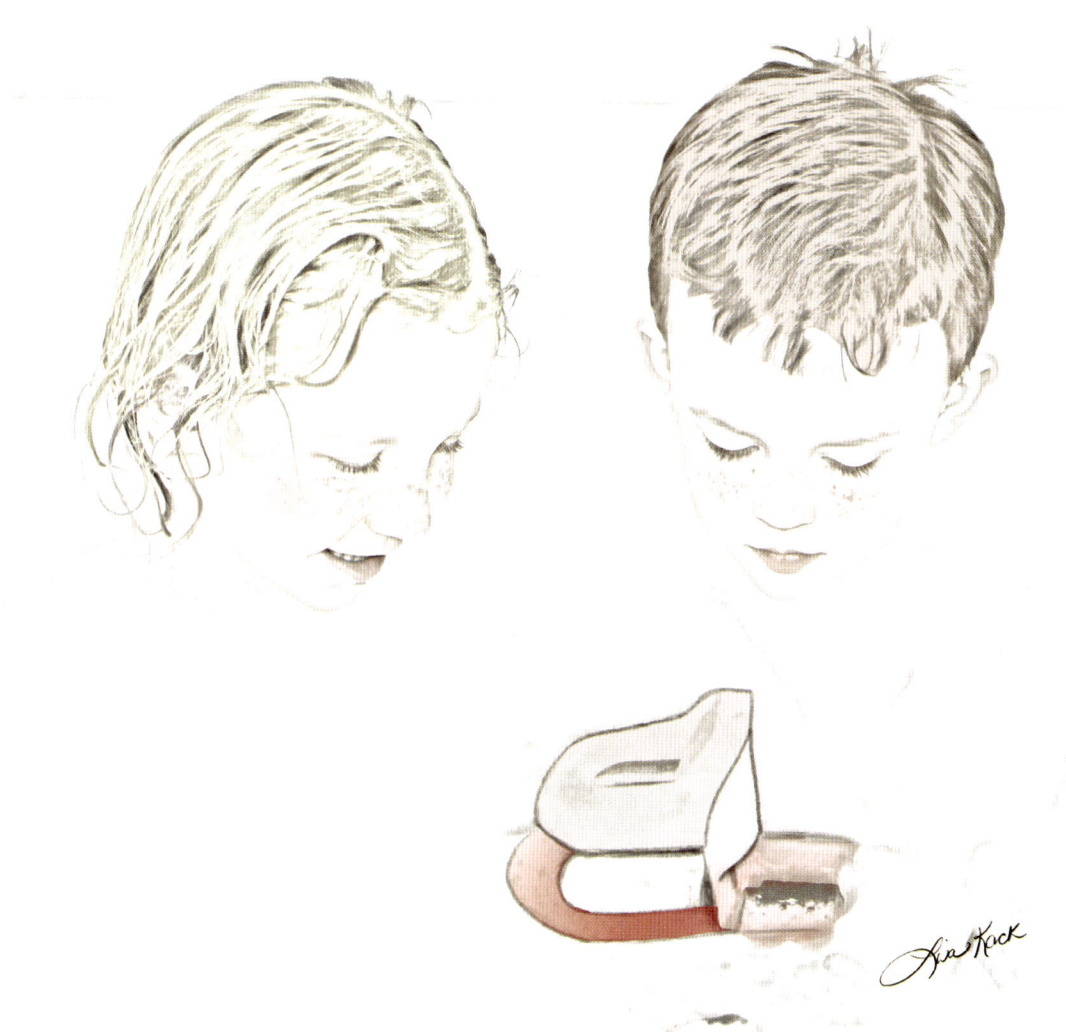

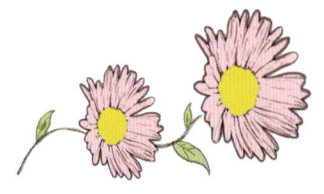

In the winter weather

When a cold draft's on the floor,

I pull my thick socks on my feet

To keep me toasty warm.

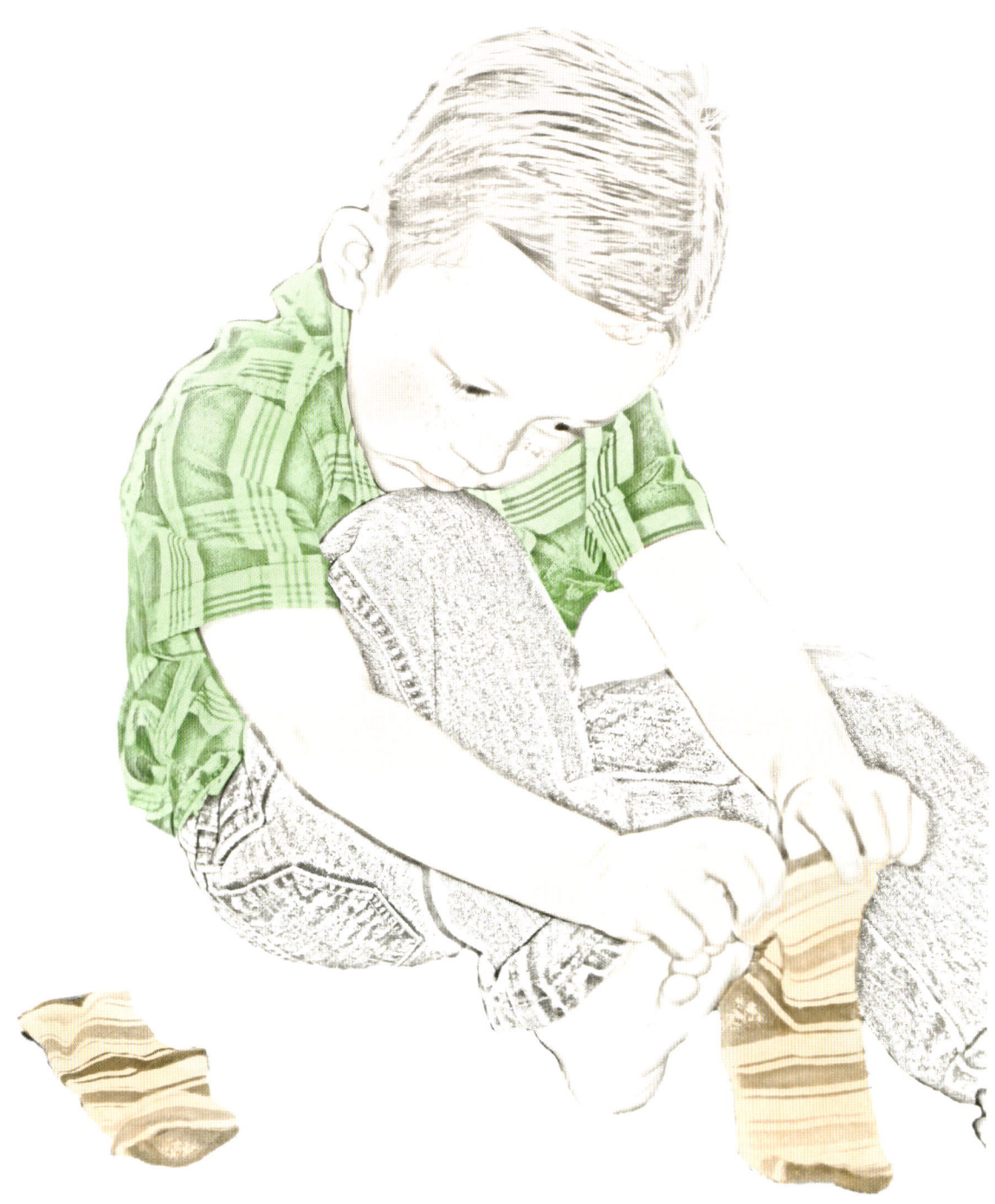

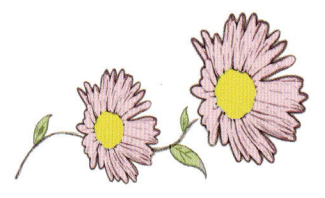

Every morning I brush my teeth

And before I go to bed.

My teeth are sparkling white

So I can give a smile bright.

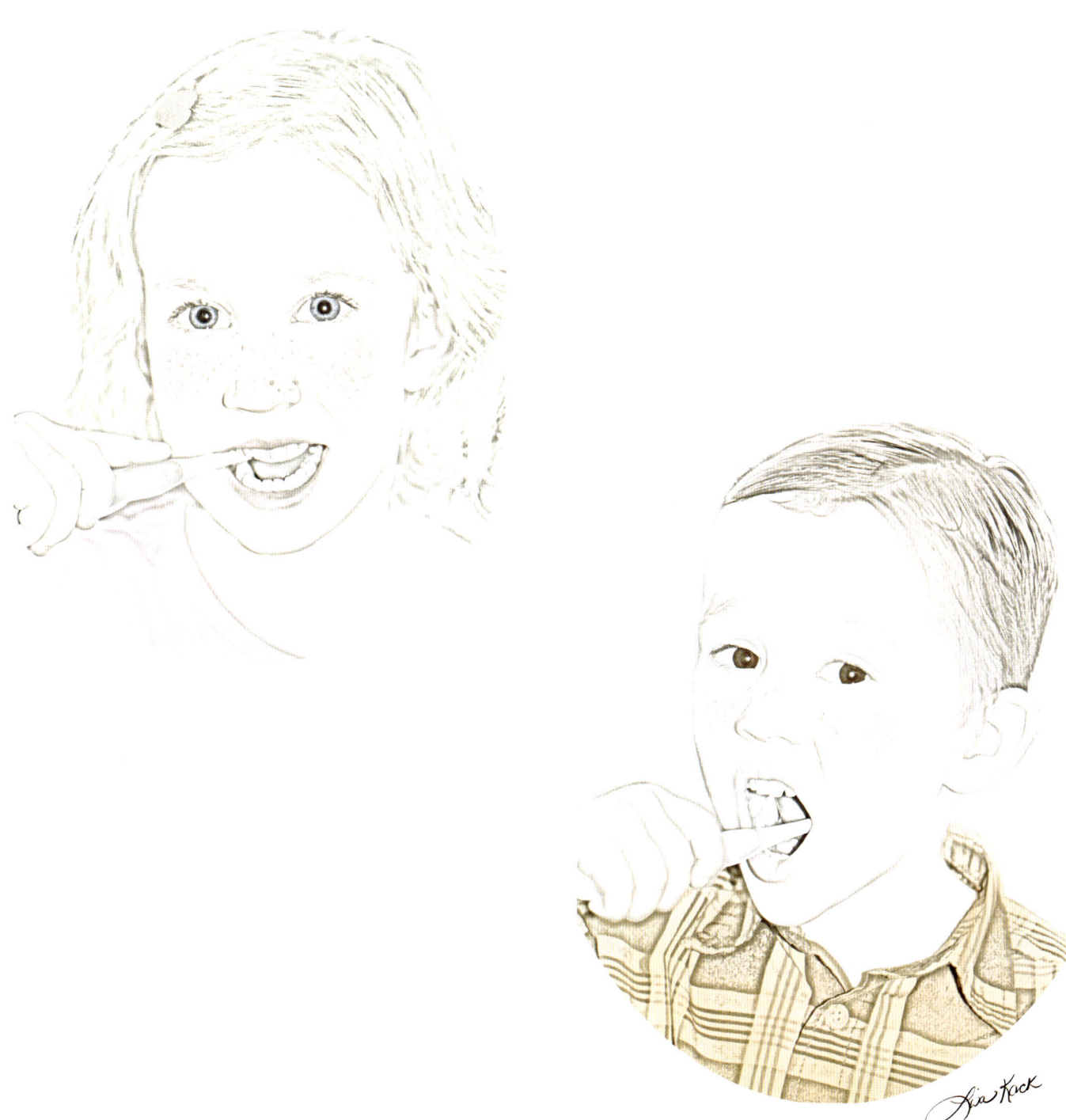

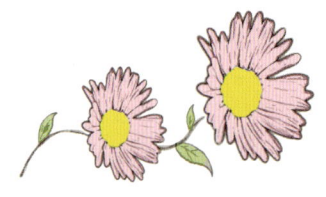

When the winter snow falls

And I go sledding on the hill,

I put my hat, coat, gloves and boots on

So I won't get a chill.

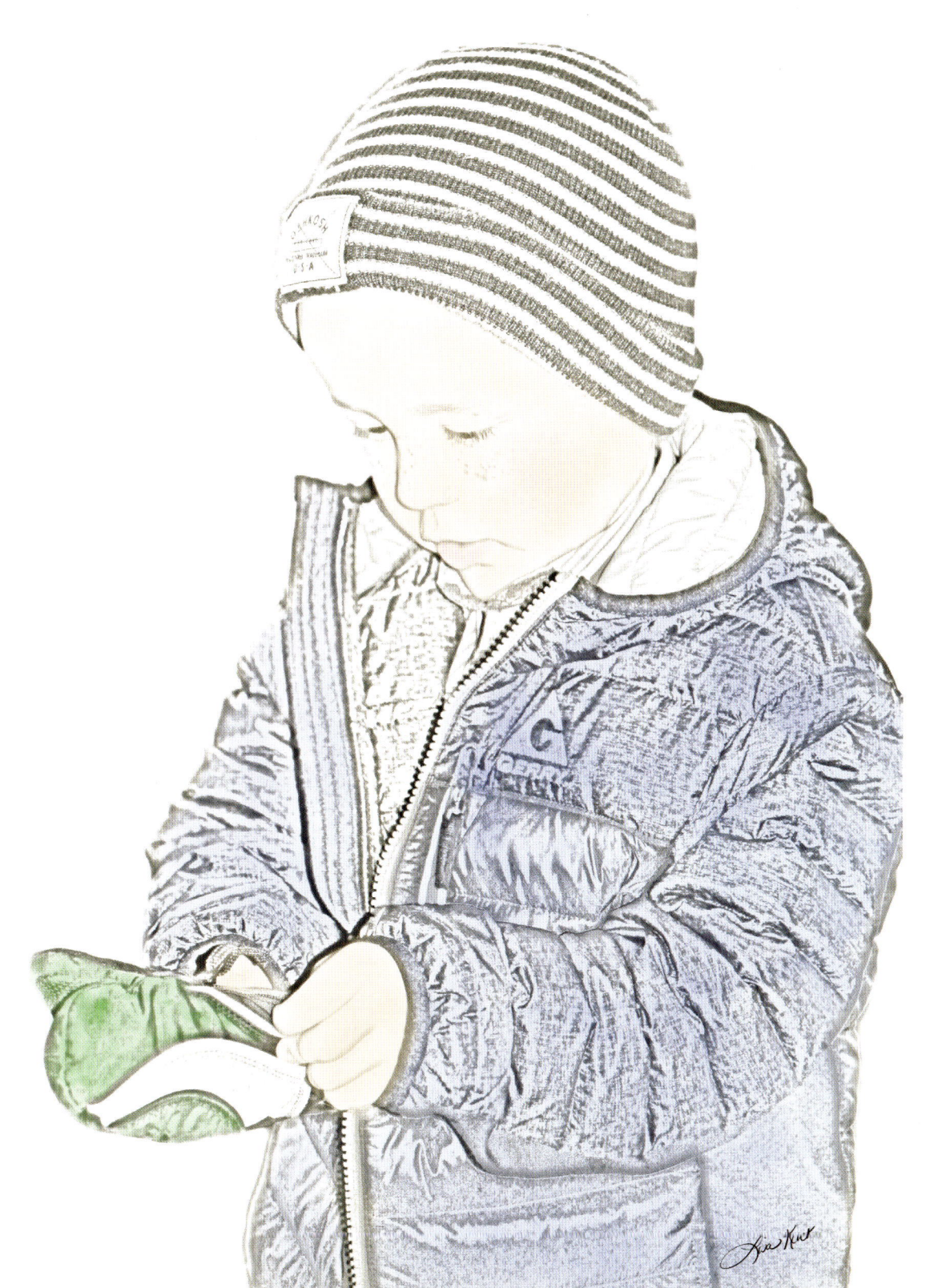

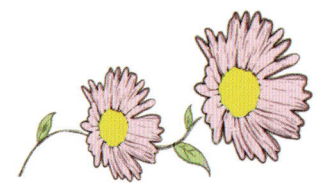

On days when I'm at school

I know one important rule:

To never touch my face

When I'm in a public place.

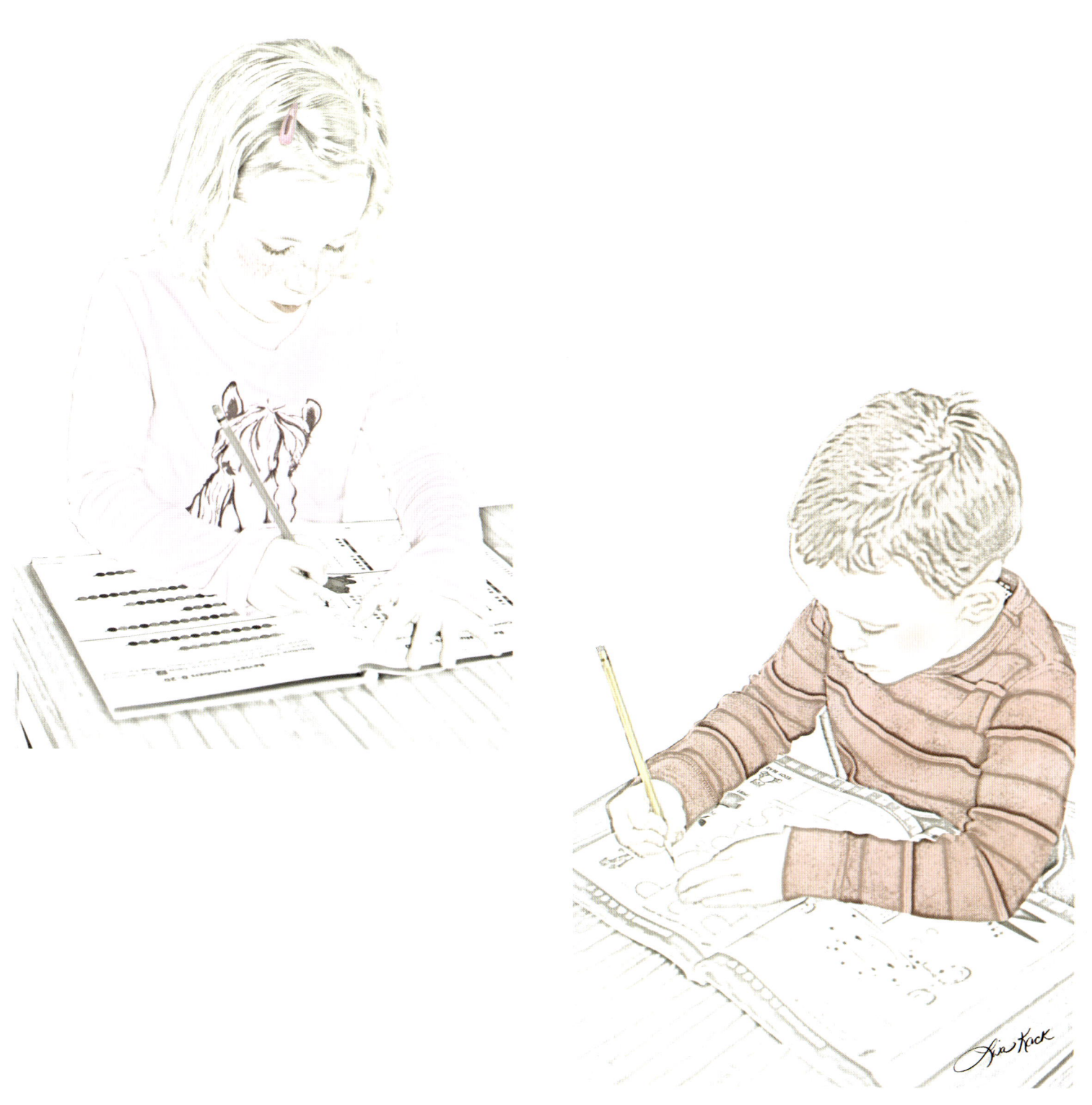

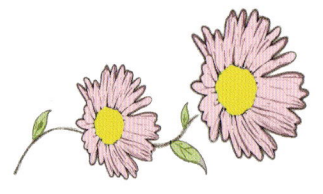

When I sit down for a meal,

I eat up all my food.

Each nutrient is stored away

For energy to run and play.

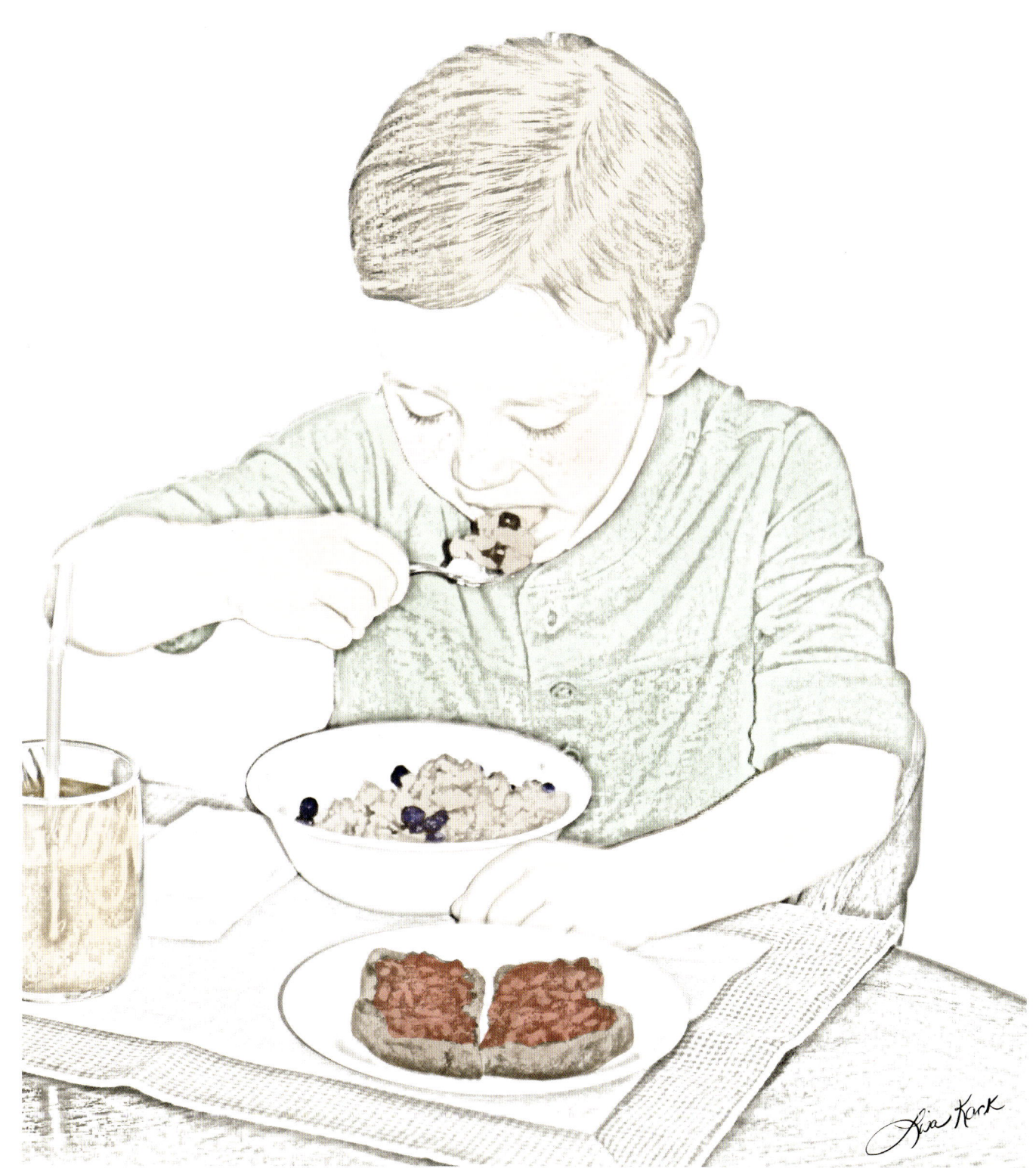

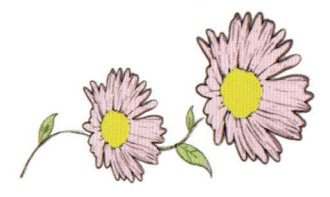

A very favorite time of day

Is when I go outside to play.

I ride my bike, explore the yard,

Throw a ball, play with my dog.

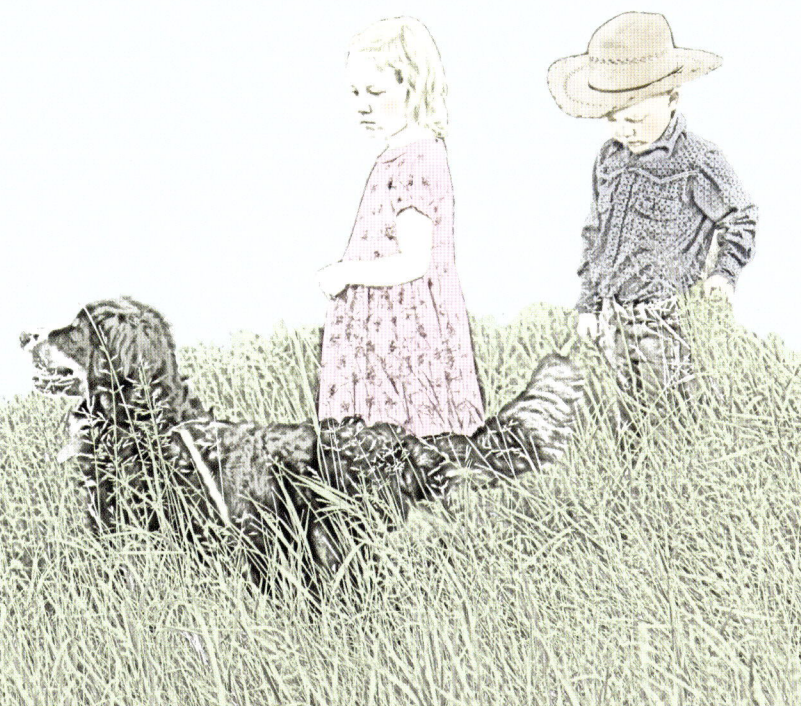

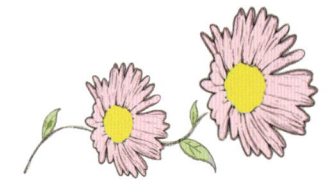

If I've done all that I can

To be a Healthy Me,

And the sniffle bug still makes me say

"A-choo,"

I make sure to cover my cough and sneeze

So others will stay well, too!

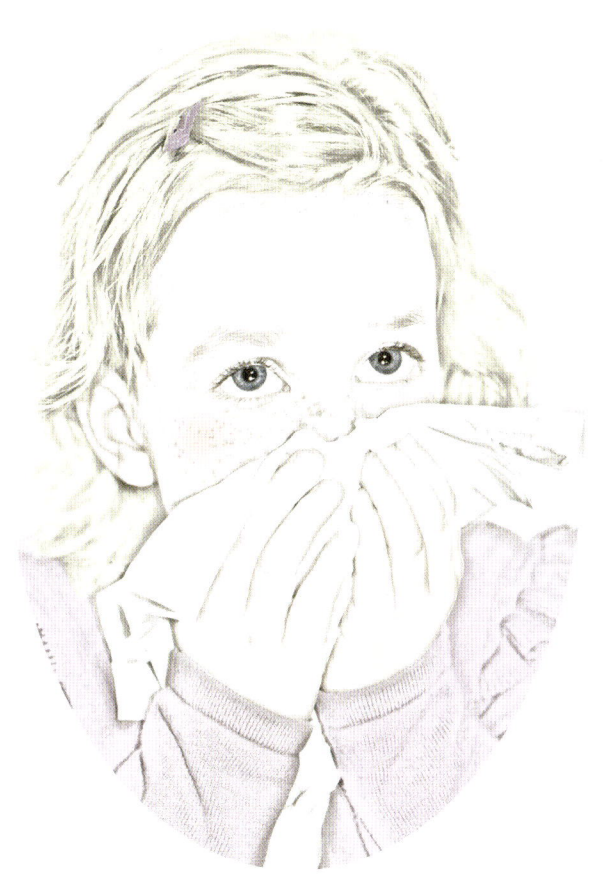
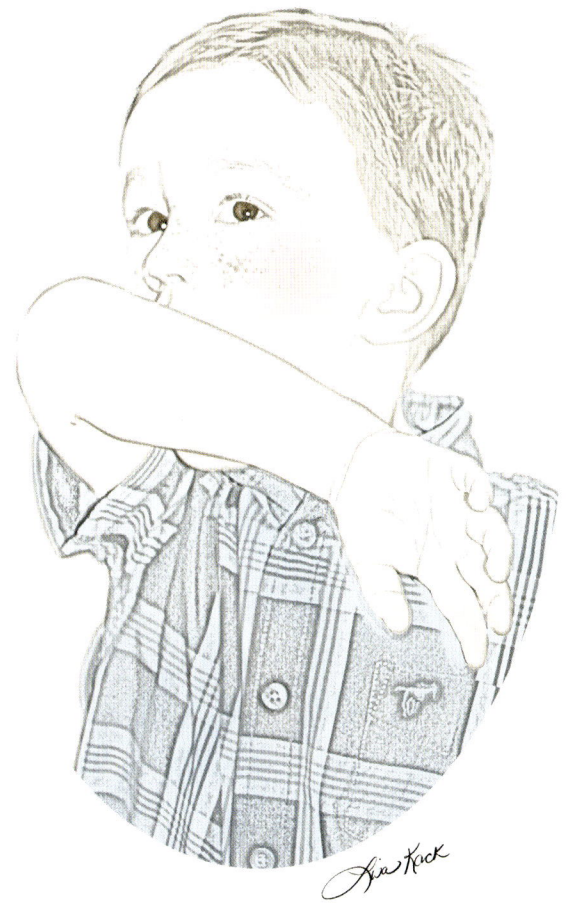

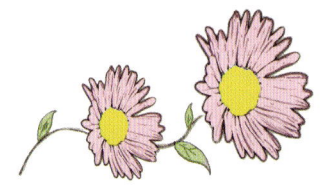

Being healthy is lots of fun

For kids like Little Me

If every day I do the things

That make a Healthy Me!

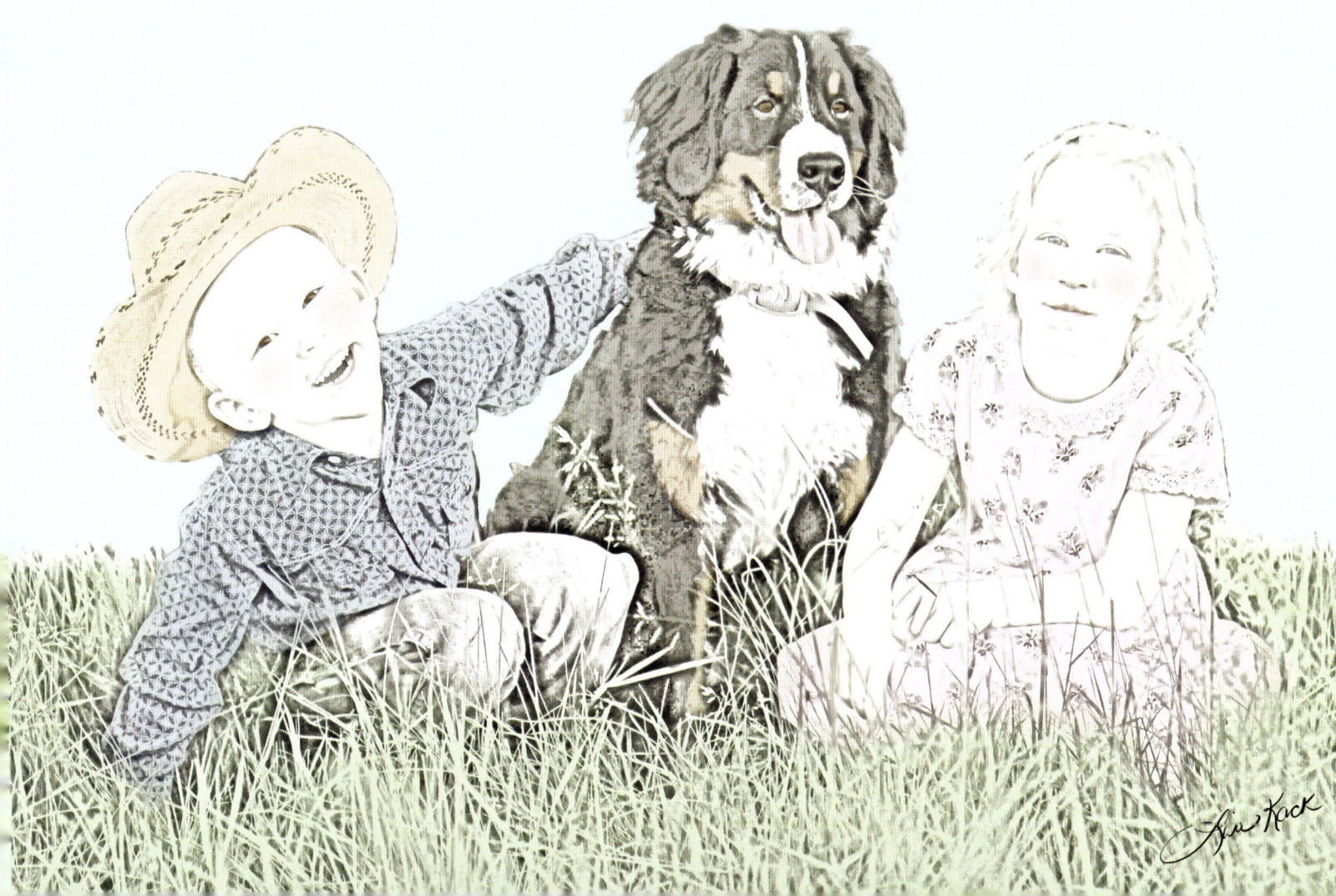

A Note From the Author:

I have had the privilege of serving as a nurse for 20 years, with experience primarily in Emergency and Intensive Care. While working I encountered diseases of varied severity in the Pediatric population and had the opportunity to observe what factors may predispose kids to illness, including the common cold.

In "A Healthy Little Me" I am sharing a collection of valuable health principles which include simple practices that kids can do every day for optimal health. Kids will enjoy reading the poetic story and learning how much fun it is to prevent illness and stay healthy!

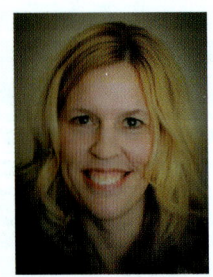 Lisa Kack, RN, BSN